Angels by the Bedside

Angels by the Bedside

Guides at the End of Life

ANNA M. ANTONOWICH RN, FNP

Caring for patients with cancer has been an honor and a blessing.

This book is dedicated to the patients, family, care-givers, and friends who have shared their incredible stories with me.

Acknowledgments

I would like to thank my family and friends for their support throughout this process. To my friends and family, thank you for taking the time to provide never-ending editing and for listening to me talk endlessly about this book. To Kim, thank you for your beautiful cover and website building and for keeping me on task. And to Karen, my Tony Robbins coach, thank you for the much-needed insights and guidance I needed to see this through. To the beautiful souls whose stories I have shared, thank you. You have enriched my life and the lives of many others who have heard your stories.

And I would be remiss if I didn't thank the angels, the guides, who helped me during this time!

Table of Contents

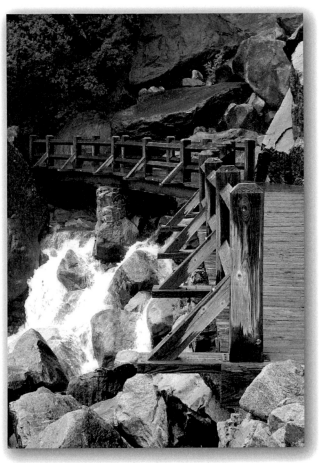

Bridgeway at Hetch Hetchy near
Wapama Falls, Yosemite, California

Introduction

Angels. Guides. Dying. Death.

This book is important for you—and for those you love and care for. It's about dying. Dying is not a topic most feel comfortable discussing. I find many people are unprepared when faced with the loss of a loved one, a friend, or a companion, especially if they have not gone through this process before. Death is a spiritual journey, one most believe is traveled alone. The stories I share will show there is a bridge on which those who have left this life return to guide those preparing to leave. They offer us hope, the reassurance that none of us are ever truly alone.

I have been at the bedsides of numerous folks before they passed away, and many have shared who was with them prior to death. They told me of the beings, or angels, who were there to guide them on that last earthly journey, a journey to the next world. Unfortunately, most won't share with friends or family because they feel they won't be believed.

I have included stories of those who have died and returned to share their experiences. Their journeys were just too valuable not to share. They give us insight into what can happen, what is possible, and why it's important to keep an open mind.

One story is of an angel presenting to the person in a dream…twice. It was a warning yet also a message of hope. Several other stories include near-death experiences in which patients have died and returned to this life.

I have found there are common threads within their stories. At the end of each story, I provide suggestions on how to be supportive during this most difficult yet precious of times. The goal is to create an atmosphere of understanding, peace, love, and hope.

This book was written with encouragement from others—family, patients, caregivers, and friends—and nudges from the angels. It is based on the observations and conversations I've had with those who were dying. Most gave me permission to share their stories. For those who did not give permission, I've changed their names and locations to protect their privacy.

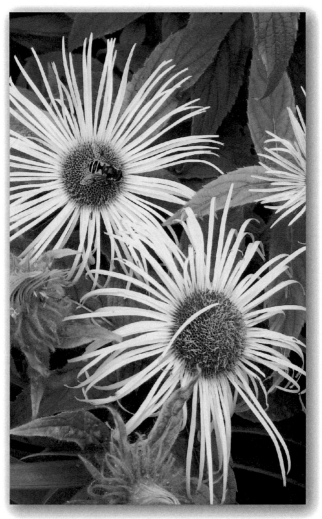

The brightness of the yellow flowers in
spring, a reminder of my mom.

One

MOM

"I'm dying. When can you get here?" my mother said calmly during an early-morning phone call.

"Are you dying now?" I asked.

"No," she said.

"I have patients to see and a few discharges to write. I can be there later this afternoon. Will that be OK?"

"Yes. I'll see you then." She then hung up the phone.

This was my first conversation of the day with my mom. She had dementia, which had worsened over the previous three years. She had lived independently until eight months prior to this call. She was diagnosed, at age eighty, with a heart condition called atrial fibrillation, which decreased the blood flow to her brain. When she was evaluated at a university hospital, we were told she had dementia with minor signs of Alzheimer's disease.

When my mom told me she was dying, I wasn't ready to believe her. Dementia could be a cruel disease, and there was a great chance she wouldn't remember the call. She knew who I was, as with most of the family. My phone number was at the top of the list, so I received daily morning calls. But this call was different. It was not her usual reorienting to her surroundings and calming herself down.

My mother had been a fairly active and happy person before her diagnosis. She worked at the local university for years and had owned a bookstore. She went to church on occasion, believed in God, and was a Christian. She also believed in aliens and flying saucers. We spent many nights during my young childhood outside watching the stars, the heavens. Her beliefs, though, would be challenged in her middle years.

When my mother was in her forties, my older brother died at the young age of twenty-one years. He had survived a tour on a riverboat in Vietnam only to be killed in a car accident a few miles from home. My mom was devastated, as any mother would be. She had lost her first-born, her only son. She searched for answers, reading books on the afterlife, most anything she could find related to the subject. She sought out pastors, psychics, palm readers, and clair-voyants. She even had a séance performed in an attempt to reconnect with my brother. She needed to know he wasn't afraid—that he was OK and in the place she had always believed was there. She needed hope.

I called her ten minutes later, feeling she would most likely have forgotten our earlier conversation.

She answered on the first ring.

"I'm dying. You'll be here this afternoon, right?"

"Yes, I'll be there."

"OK. See you then."

Holy cow.

Mom was not on pain medications or anything that would make her hallucinate. I knew she hadn't taken something to make her confused. She had slept well and had been active the day prior.

As a nurse practitioner and an oncology nurse for years, I believed her. I quickly called my sister and niece and informed them of what she said. They asked if I knew when she was going to die. Well, no. I didn't. But I believed her.

Later that day, I arrived to find her looking a little tired. She was outside talking with her brother, sister-in-law, and cousins. Mom had been doing well up until that point, despite residing in an assisted-living facility due to her dementia. I had placed her on hospice almost six months prior knowing her dementia was worsening. But hospice was going to drop her from their program in just a few days as she was doing so well.

When I had a couple of minutes alone with her, I asked, "Mom, who has been with you?"

"Charles Ray."

Charles Ray was my brother who had passed away in 1971. Uh-oh.

"You must be so excited to see him after so long."

"I am."

"Mom, what does he do with you during his visits?"

"He walks in the halls with me. He sits with me while I eat. He talks with me."

"How wonderful. How long has he been with you?"

"Two weeks." Again, uh-oh.

Then, in a rather stern voice, she asked me what I thought it all meant.

"You said you are dying, and he's here to go with you," I replied.

"Oh." And that was the last she mentioned of his visits.

She continued to go about her daily activities, but she was slowing down, eating little. She slept more during the day. Fatigue came more easily if she was up and about. She didn't want to leave the facility she was living in, even for short trips to go for a drive about town.

Later that week, as friends and family made their way to her, so did the hospice nurse. She had come to close my mom's case. The nurse felt my mom was doing well, had put on weight, was eating well, and was active. My mom never mentioned that she knew who the nurse was, never remembering the weekly visits. The nurse informed my mom she would not be coming any longer as she was doing so well. My mom's reply was that she "shouldn't close her case because it would just need to be opened again soon, and you'll have to do all that paperwork again." After many discussions with the nurse and her administrator, my mom was allowed to stay on hospice.

Later the following week, an uncanny event occurred. I was sitting in a recliner near my mom, who was now bedridden. Miss Kitty, my mother's rather large cat, was sleeping at the foot of her bed. It was just the three of us; the rest of the family had taken a break. Quite suddenly, Miss Kitty jumped from the bed, ran to one of the corners of the room, and began howling and scratching at the wall. She then ran to another corner and repeated her behavior. Turning, she ran over to me, to the chair I was sitting in, and continued the crazy yowling and scratching. I didn't move an inch and could barely breathe! Almost as abruptly as she'd begun, she jumped back onto my mom's bed, curled up, and went back to sleep. It took minutes before I could move. I have heard of animals gravitating to people who would soon die or watching invisible things in the room, but I hadn't ever witnessed this type of behavior myself!

Animals are more sensitive than people and have heightened awareness. They see things we don't. They sense impending death. Most of us have all heard of the cat in a convalescent home going to someone prior to their death. Miss Kitty was standing guard. She definitely wasn't chasing a bug or spider as she went on her rant around my mom's room. She was making one last effort to keep her "mom" in this world.

Fourteen days after her phone call to me, my mother passed away. We weren't sure of the cause of death, only that her physical condition declined, and she passed away peacefully.

There are several learning opportunities from this experience. While it can be difficult, clarify what you hear. By taking the time to call her back, my mom confirmed she was going to die. Even with dementia, at times, they can be clear of thought and speech. I also encourage you to ask who is in the room. In most cases, they have been seeing someone, may be talking to someone but not comfortable discussing the visions unless asked in a supportive environment. There is the perception that the visions will not be taken seriously or may be considered a side effect of medication. Keeping an open mind and being observant of the less obvious will guide you further. As with the behavior of Miss Kitty, things happen. We tend to be caught up in our own sorrow and miss these precious events.

Your experiences and thoughts. How could a situation you have been involved in been improved? What would have made the situation go more smoothly?

_____

_____

_____

_____

_____

_____

_____

_____

_____

_____

_____

_____

_____

_____

_____

_____

_____

Notes

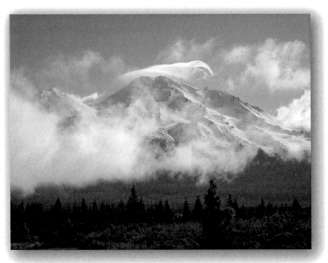
Mount Shasta, her calm before the storm.

Two

Tom

"I want to go home. I would like to go today," Tom said.

"I'm waiting on a call from your surgeon. The paperwork has been completed. I just need the final OK from your doc."

"I really want to go home," he said again, with more emphasis.

"Yes, I know. It'll be great to be home for Thanksgiving! You have an appointment on Monday with your surgeon to go over options for surgery."

I was visiting with a patient I was readying for discharge. Tom's wife and daughter-in-law were at the bedside. He commented numerous times he wanted to go home. It was the day before Thanksgiving, and Tom lived in a small town fifty miles away. It was looking like the weather was changing rapidly, and the longer it took to discharge him, the better his chances of driving home in the snow.

His son was also visiting with us, but he needed to take a phone call and have a cigarette. Tom's son had mentioned how difficult his father's illness had been on him and how it had taken him by surprise. He was having a rough time. He lived out of state and had only come to town this morning to see his father.

Tom, his wife, his daughter-in-law, and I were reviewing the possibility of surgical intervention in the near future. We talked of their family plans for the holiday. I mentioned how wonderful it would be for Tom to sleep at home, in his own bed, before dealing with what might lie ahead. At times such as these, the patients and families will ask a variety of questions. Somehow the subject of angels came up.

"Anna has a few angel stories. Would you like to hear them?" Angela said to her father-in-law.

"Sure," he said.

He asked if I knew of people seeing angels. I responded that yes, I had. So we talked of angels, the guides, who appeared by the bedside prior to death. I mentioned that patients knew who the angels were, as they were usually someone from their past.

"Anna, if we are supposed to know our angels, why am I surrounded by children, these angels, but I don't know any of them?" he asked as he pointed to the corner of the room.

"Well, we can't see them, so you will have to ask them who they are," I replied.

"Hmm. OK," he said softly.

This was not a typical comment related to guides by the bedside. My thoughts were still on the current discharge plan, to get him home for the holiday and back into town for his appointment on Monday. I was standing at the foot of his hospital bed. His wife was sitting on one side, his daughter-in-law, the other.

A minute or so later, after he mentioned the children surrounding him, he looked up at me.

"Uh-oh..." he said quietly.

The tumor, located in the back of his tongue and throat, broke open, and he began to bleed. This caught me totally off guard as I was expecting him to go home. Now, he was bleeding out of control! I knew there was nothing I could do to stop the bleeding. His daughter-in-law quickly placed a trash can under his chin to catch his blood; his wife stood at his side stroking his hair, whispering to him calmly. I panicked, ran out the door to get the nurse, ordered morphine, and incorrectly called a "code blue." He was listed as a "do not resuscitate," which means he did not wish for heroic interventions in an event such as this. The "code blue" was canceled. He was given morphine, though he would most likely not feel the effects.

He passed away quickly, within minutes.

Once the nurses had cleaned up the small amount of blood that had spilled onto the bed and gently washed Tom's face, things calmed down. His wife and daughter-in-law had remained at the bedside throughout everything. I was a mess, but they were calmer than I expected. Watching someone bleed out can be horrific at best, yet they were, through their tears, very calm. The social worker and chaplain were called to provide assistance.

"This was very sudden. I'm so sorry he passed this way. But I have to ask: You were both pretty calm while this was happening. Why?" I asked.

"He had angels with him. He wasn't alone," his wife replied.

Then, the patient's son returned to the room. He was shocked to find his father had passed.

"I shouldn't have taken the call. I should have stayed in the room! I feel so awful," he said.

"Your dad made this choice on some level. It was an intense time, and maybe he chose to have you not witness his death. You were here to see him, and that is what mattered," I said in response.

My patient had told me repeatedly he "wanted to go home." I wasn't prepared for home to be heaven. In my mind, I was discharging him to go home to be with his family for Thanksgiving, to be sleeping in his own bed, getting ready for the next step in his disease treatment.

Pay close attention to what the patient, or the person dying, is saying. Most of the time they will give us clues. If we are fortunate, they will even tell us when they will pass.

We, as providers, are sometimes so focused on 'our ' plan we fail to listen, truly listen, to what is right in front of us. Patients do seem to 'choose' who will be with them at the time of death. I've seen a loved one step out for a much needed cup of coffee or to answer a call and the patient dies. A patient may wait until someone from out of town arrives before they will die. While we all wish we could be with a loved one, to share the patient's last breath, it may not be in the ultimate plan.

Your experiences and thoughts. How could a situation you have been involved in been improved? What would have made the situation go more smoothly?

_____

_____

_____

_____

_____

_____

_____

_____

_____

_____

_____

_____

_____

_____

_____

_____

_____

Notes

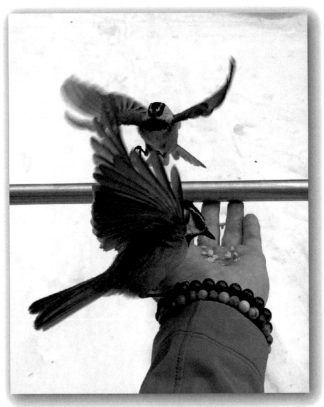

Chicadees in winter. The visitors who traveled with us on our journey.

Three

"They're out there," George said anxiously. We looked around his room, finding no one there. No one.

"Who?"

"My dad and Karen."

I was the charge nurse on a busy hematology/oncology/transplant unit. George's call light had come on. It was a call from the patient's bathroom, which usually meant the patient had fallen or, worse yet, was injured. As the patient's nurse and I ran down the hall toward the patient's room, many thoughts were running through our minds. We were going through all the possibilities for why the light was on. We were hoping he wasn't lying on the floor in a puddle of blood. We were preparing for the worst.

We entered the room and opened the door to the bathroom. Much to our surprise, George was standing there, not bleeding, uninjured, fully awake, and oriented. He looked a little apprehensive.

George had leukemia. We had treated his disease, but it had returned and was growing rapidly. All of his family had passed, and there were no close friends to care for him in his last days, thus making him ineligible for hospice. He was admitted to the hospital to pass away with dignity and without pain. George was expected to pass away in a matter of days. At the time, he was able to walk, continued to eat small amounts of food, and was not in pain. But he was afraid to die, especially alone.

We knew his dad had passed away many years ago. Karen, who had been one of our nurses, died just six months prior to this admission. Karen had provided his primary nursing care, beginning with his diagnosis until the time she herself became too ill to work.

"Well, I believe they can come in here," I said.

"What do I do?" George said, continuing to sound a bit frazzled at having these beings in his room.

"Maybe ask them why they are here."

I had never suggested someone, let alone a patient, talk with beings they couldn't see. Something inside guided me to these words, which would change the way I viewed the experience of dying to this day. He was not receiving pain medicine or other drugs that would make him hallucinate. We believed what he was telling us.

"Are you afraid of them? Are they scary?" I asked.

"No," he replied as he cautiously stepped out of the bathroom.

"Will you be OK alone?"

"Yes, I think so."

"If you need us, just use the call light, and we'll come back as quickly as we can."

As George walked into his room, he did so slowly, looking about. He lay back in the hospital bed. Sunlight was streaming through the window into his room. He was not afraid of these beings—had he been, we would not have left him alone. Once we stepped out the room, he asked his dad and Karen why they were there. They informed him that no one ever dies alone. They were there to "go with him, to guide him." Karen and George's dad were waiting patiently for him to begin the dying process. They had come for him. Over time, George became more comfortable with his guests. After a while, he seemed filled with happiness at seeing Karen and his father. It was wonderful to observe the changes in George's acceptance of dying, his movement from anxiousness to calm.

For George, he knew there was more to life and there was a life after death. He died at peace, in his sleep, without pain or fear, knowing he was not alone.

⌒

As nurses we are problem solvers, especially when it comes to a possible emergency. It took a minute to realize the situation we were walking into, the situation we were privileged to be a part of. We needed to switch from an urgent situation to that of a nurturing one. Again, asking the patient or loved one questions regarding the beings is key. Providing a safe environment and encouraging the patient talk with the beings will give them a sense of control in these situations. We can provide reassurance to the patient they are seeing the beings and they are truly there. For the patient, these beings are real.

I also ask if the patient is afraid of the bedside visitors. I am not aware of anyone who was visited by an angel who brings about fear. These beings bring peace. If the patient states they are frightened by the visitors, this should be discussed with the patient's nurses or physician as it may be an issue with medications, physiologic changes, or changes due to their disease.

From the time of his first mentioning he had visitors, when I entered the room I asked if they were present and where they were in the room. We cannot see them so asking is necessary even if it feels uncomfortable. I also didn't want to accidently sit on or walk through one of the beings! By showing acceptance of the situation the patient's anxiety is lessened.

Your experiences and thoughts. How could a situation you have been involved in been improved? What would have made the situation go more smoothly?

_____

_____

_____

_____

_____

_____

_____

_____

_____

_____

_____

_____

_____

_____

_____

_____

_____

_____

_____

_____

Notes

Notes

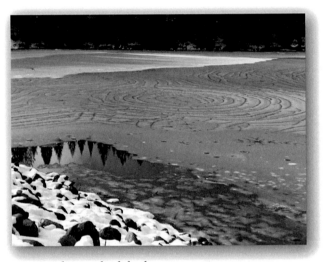

Circles in the lake between winter storms.
The connectedness of life and death.

Four

"Hi, Anna-min."

"Hi, Pall. I hear your mother has been here," I said.

"Yes, she has!" Pall said clearly, which caught me a bit by surprise.

"How wonderful! It's been a long time since you've seen her," I replied.

"I know. It has."

My ex-father-in-law, Pall, had been diagnosed with hydrocephalus a year prior to this conversation. It is a condition related to the imbalance of cerebrospinal fluid (CSF) in the brain. Normally, as CSF is produced, it should also be drained. A consistent pressure in the brain is maintained. But with hydrocephalus, the fluid is not draining as fast as it is being produced, causing increased pressure on the brain. This condition created progressive dementia-like symptoms in a man who had been very active. In the past, he had loved to play golf and snow ski. For the past year, even with a shunt placed to help regulate the pressure, he became increasingly disabled. He had not spoken much in the past six months. He was unable to walk without assistance. Sometimes he was combative. Most of the time, he was confused.

He was admitted to the hospital with pneumonia but this time was not in the intensive care unit. He was not receiving pain medication or any new medications other than antibiotics. I had come to see him, given my long history in the family. My ex-husband, Danni, told me of Pall, saying he had seen his mother in his hospital room earlier that day. Pall's mom had passed away many, many years ago in Iceland. When I heard that he'd seen her, I knew what was coming. He was seeing someone who had passed away, someone who was there to go with him.

I asked Pall directly and confirmed he was seeing his own mother. After he talked to me, he went silent again. The mood in the hospital room was somber. All eyes were on me. His adult children were in the room, as was my ex-mother-in-law, Asta. There was tension in the room. Pall's illness was bringing up many issues within the family. The doctor had mentioned hospice, but some family members were not yet ready to move in that direction. They wanted the antibiotics to work and Pall to continue to live as long as he could. Knowing there were conflicting ideas regarding the next step in Pall's care, I spoke up. I knelt down in front of Asta, taking her hands in mine.

"Asta, what do you think Pall would want?" I asked through the tears pooling in my eyes. "You know what his seeing his mom means."

"I do. He didn't want to keep doing this. He said last year he did not want any more treatments, no more hospital," Asta answered.

"Would you like to take him home? Or would you like to have him stay here until he passes?"

"I would like to take him home. He would want to be home," Asta said through her tears. She would be taking her love home for the last time.

It was a difficult day with very difficult conversations. To acknowledge an impending death, to know the end is near, is so sad for everyone. Pall was a vibrant, happy man through most of his life. His blue eyes would sparkle so brightly, and his joy was infectious. His love of skiing brought him such happiness. Pall's life on earth was moving quickly to an end. His mother was there to go with him, to guide him to the other side.

Pall was discharged to go home the next day. His wife and children shared in his care. He passed away peacefully almost a week later.

⁓

Even with family, listening for the clues is important. After months of unclear speech and confusion, Pall was talking, though it was for a very limited time. Many of the dying may have an animated, energized period shortly before they pass. These episodes may be misunderstood, giving false hope that the loved one is improving and may not die. While there can be miracles, most often, this period of time is short lived and the patient continues their decline.

Look to the current decision maker in the family. In this case it was Asta, his love, his wife, his best friend, and mother of his children. Thankfully, Asta had already discussed with Pall his wishes while he was capable of expressing them. She had talked with him and knew what he had wanted. At times like this, supporting a decision may be difficult but it is necessary for unity and peace for the dying and those left behind. Making the decision to stop a potential life saving treatment or therapy is difficult. Knowing what someone would like to do takes the decision making off family or friends and allows the patient the ultimate control of the situation.

There may be differing opinions regarding the course and goals of care. Passing away peacefully, without pain or with only minimal pain, without feeling air hunger, are most people's goals. Shifting from full care and treatment to hospice care, the goals change. Care changes. The focus moves to that of comfort. This can be a scary time for someone not exposed to this type of situation in the past. Many things may be said out of fear or anger, from a sense of loss of control. Clear communication, allowing everyone to vocalize their opinions, can be healing, but needs to be done from a place of love and respect for each other.

Your experiences and thoughts. How could a situation you have been involved in been improved? What would have made the situation go more smoothly?

_____

_____

_____

_____

_____

_____

_____

_____

_____

_____

_____

_____

_____

_____

_____

_____

_____

_____

Notes

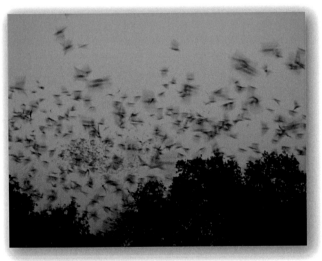

Night sky filled with bats taking flight.
While death may be chaotic for some,
there is a pattern to the path.

Five

Katie was a twenty-five-year-old diagnosed with lymphoma. She was found to have masses in her chest on a chest x-ray. The x-ray was part of the physical exam required for her application to the police academy. Her dream was to have a career and be able to support her family. Her husband and their two children were out of the country, staying with her in-laws. Her husband had been severely injured and was paralyzed from the waist down several years ago and required more help than Katie could provide. He and the children moved to his homeland in Central America, where there was family to care for them. The plan was for Katie's family to reunite once her police training was complete.

Katie had the required scans and tests done. Chemotherapy was ordered, and she started down the treatment path and put her career plans on hold.

She did not have much social support. In her words, her family was "a bit dysfunctional." She was not able to rely on them. She was very clear that she did not want their help. Katie did the best she could with the few friends she had. After multiple cycles of various chemotherapy regimens, scans showed her disease was growing with a vengeance. She didn't have long to live.

She was devastated.

She did not want to leave. She did not want to die. She missed her family. Katie then realized she wasn't going to see her children or her husband again in this lifetime.

As there weren't locally reliable family members or friends who could take time from work to care for her at home, Katie was admitted to the hospital. She would remain with us until she passed away. She was a fighter, determined to give it her all in the hopes of a miracle. As her health declined and she became more ill, we had many heart-to-heart talks. Katie shared stories about her children, whom she missed desperately. She missed her husband.

During this most difficult time, she continued to severely mistrust her blood relatives. They rarely saw her and hadn't offered to care for her when she needed it during her treatment. Katie was concerned they would try to take her children away from their father. She did not want them notified when she died.

I was her nurse the day she passed away. As she was without a caregiver, I was in the room as much as possible. I noticed Katie would suddenly open her eyes, and they would occasionally track around the room as if she were watching someone moving about. She would put her hands up like she was fending someone off. Then, as if someone were reaching for her, she would withdraw her arms. She would pull away, retracting into a small ball with her tired, thin body.

She was alone when she passed toward the end of my shift.

I entered the room to find she had thrown up as she took her last breath. There was no evidence of a seizure or another situation to explain the vomiting. It was as if she were fighting for her life. Katie had not wanted to leave, was not ready to go. And now she had died without someone from this world at her bedside. But it seemed she did have guides, the beings who were there to go with her, even though she hadn't wanted to go.

Several hours later, as I ended my shift, I informed the night charge nurse what I knew, and I told her that the patient had requested that her family not be allowed to take her belongings or see her once she passed.

I started my long drive home. After fifteen minutes, I had an overwhelming urge to call the charge nurse. Something, a strong pull in me, made me pull over to make the call. It was before cell phones were popular, so I had to find a pay phone. The next off-ramp was in a rather seedy part of town and very scary, but the urge to call was intense.

All I kept hearing was "Don't let them take my children. Don't let them take my things."

As I pulled off the freeway, all I could think of was Katie. Her children and husband meant the world to her. The pay phone was at a gas station, so I would be outside, in the dark…alone. But I knew, deep down, I would be safe.

I phoned the night charge nurse at the hospital. Katie's family had shown up, having heard from someone that she might have passed. They were asking for her belongings. I told the nurse why I called and let her know that they were not to have her things.

The family was turned away, and social services were notified.

Not everyone is ready to leave this earth for a variety of reasons. The guides seemed to be there yet she did not want to leave with them, was not ready to go. So she fought them. The sadness surrounding this type of situation does not fade easily.

Patient's fears should be honored not discounted. She was afraid for her children. HIPPA regulations prohibit us now from discussing a patient's health or death unless there is written permission. As providers, we try to work with our patients to make sure their wishes are known. She had taken steps to assure her children would remain with their father, and designated a friend to handle her affairs after she passed. But even with her children safe, she had worried her family would somehow take her children. At the time of Katie's death, we honored her wishes as she had asked. Her family was turned away.

Pay attention to the messages we see, feel and hear after someone passes. I've asked those who were open to it, that they make contact after they cross over. They can let someone know they are ok in ways the earthbound person will understand. Sometimes it is with familiar scents, the sensation of touch, an angelic vision or visitation, hearing or seeing them in dreams. With Katie, I felt strongly that I needed to make the call to the charge nurse after I left the hospital and I honored the request. While it was a bit scary and I thought the charge nurse might think I was just very tired after a long shift, I did what was asked of me. I've never regretted making the call. Sometimes we just need to trust we are doing the right thing and follow the push we are feeling.

Your experiences and thoughts. How could a situation you have been involved in been improved? What would have made the situation go more smoothly?

_____

_____

_____

_____

_____

_____

_____

_____

_____

_____

_____

_____

_____

_____

_____

_____

_____

Notes

Notes

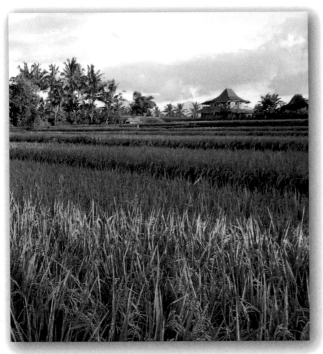

The beauty and unexpected peacefulness
of the rice fields in Bali.

Six

"Anna, I'm not afraid to die." Doc said in soft, tired voice

These were the first words my close friend said to me on the phone from the ICU.

He had recently undergone heart surgery. A few days postop, while walking in the hallway of the ICU, he "coded." His heart went into an erratic rhythm, and subsequently, he went into cardiac arrest. Dropping to the floor, he died. As medical personnel were resuscitating him, he went on a journey.

"You heard what happened," he said quietly.

"Yes," I said.

"I sat next to God. I'm not afraid to die."

He had survived two different cancer diagnoses and treatments during this life. Now he was recovering from heart surgery. He was young, only in his midfifties. He watched his health slip, becoming more and more disabled over time. Due to poor health, he had to give up his medical practice. He wished for a miracle, but he was a practical man. He understood his health was poor and time could be limited. His love for his children was immense, which made his declining health even more upsetting. At this point he was unable to do so many of the things that most fathers enjoy doing with their kids: going for long walks, teaching them to ride bicycles, playing in the yard…simple things.

My friend had not been a religious man. At times, he was a bit angry with God or with his perception of life's guiding forces. To add to the complexity of his life, he had gone through a messy divorce. It had been a difficult time for him.

"When can you get here?" he asked.

"I have to work this week but can be there this weekend. Will that be OK? Or do I need to come now?"

"This weekend is OK. I want to talk with you more about what happened, about the journey I went on."

That Friday, I flew up to see him. As I entered his room in the ICU, he looked tired, but something had changed.

"Anna, I sat next to God," he informed me again, this time face to face. He seemed so at peace.

Coming from a man who hadn't believed much in religion, let alone God, this was another surprise, even though he had told me the same thing earlier in the week. He told me of his experience of going to heaven. He said it was filled with overwhelming love, enveloping him in warmth and compassion. It was peaceful. He sat next to God. He said they spoke for quite some time. He was told it was not yet his time to leave his earthbound life. He still had things to do.

Again, he told me, "I'm not afraid to die."

He began to recover slowly. He was finally able to be transferred to the rehabilitation center, to begin the long journey toward living independently. He missed his dog, his home. He knew he needed to build his strength physically to be able to go home.

During this period of recovery, he spent time with his kids, his friends, and his colleagues. Much to the surprise of all of us, he also made peace with his ex-wife!

After a couple of weeks in rehab, his health again declined. He was readmitted to the ICU. Recovery was not likely. His illness, this time, would take him. He was going to die.

I left work and began the long drive to see him one last time. I was going to overnight at a friend's house, when I spoke with one of his doctors, who was also a dear friend of mine. Time was moving swiftly. I would most likely not make it in time to see my friend before he passed.

Traveling after a long day at work soon caught up with me. Once in bed, I fell asleep quickly. I had been sleeping soundly when I was suddenly awakened. I heard his voice. I slowly opened my eyes, and there he was, standing at the foot of my bed. I glanced at the clock: 3:20 a.m. I closed my eyes, but I could still see him and continued to hear his voice. He was healthy in appearance, with a glow around him. He talked with me, telepathically, a type of mind meld. My friend spoke of his journey and how appreciative he was to have had his time on earth, for his friends and family. He again talked of how truly amazing it was, the world beyond the one we know here on earth.

He was OK and not afraid. He was at peace. We said our good-byes, and he was gone. Much to my amazement, the dog that was sleeping with me on the bed did not stir. I looked at the clock again. Twenty minutes had passed.

Wow! I knew I was awake as I could feel my heart pounding. I was definitely awake!

Later that morning, I phoned his sister, who wasn't able to be at his bedside prior to his passing either. I asked her if anything odd had happened to her the night prior.

"He visited you too?" she said rather surprised.

"Yes, he did." And we shared our stories with one another.

As he had with me earlier that morning, he also visited with his sister. He visited her at 3:00 a.m., just before his visit with me. The focus of the conversation was very similar, his appearance the same. From what we later learned, we were the only ones he visited prior to his physical death.

I know he is with God, surrounded by love and happiness.

⌒⟶

Try to be open to what is happening in front of you. Listen to what the dying are telling you. Situations may present themselves, such as the nighttime visit from my friend. They may come to us in our dreams. Other times, it may be unspoken, yet we know. Our friends and loved ones do not always present themselves after they move on, so do not be discouraged. They may be in such a wonderful place and they have moved on.

Unfinished business may keep the dying from moving on. Once these issues are resolved or even attended to, it will be time for them to leave. We have all heard of the patient waiting for someone to come to the bedside. They pass away after the person or persons have come to see them. At other times, it can be after they're told it's ok to go, to die. As hard as this is for those of us left behind, the dying may need to hear we will miss them but we will be ok.

Your experiences and thoughts. How could a situation you have been involved in been improved? What would have made the situation go more smoothly?

_____

_____

_____

_____

_____

_____

_____

_____

_____

_____

_____

_____

_____

_____

_____

_____

_____

Notes

Notes

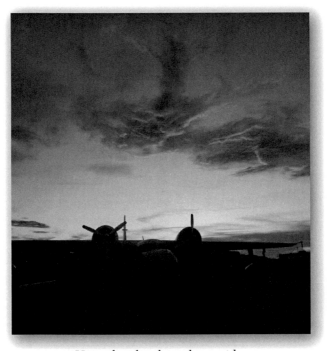

Her pilot, her love, her guide.

Seven

"I don't want to be a military wife this time," Greta said as she reached out.

Greta was a widow but was always surrounded by family. She had been married to a career military man who had passed away some time ago.

Greta was diagnosed with leukemia in her later years. Her life expectancy was not long; it was only a matter of months. Greta wanted to stay alive as long as possible.

She and her family were seeing me for palliative care. She was not placed on hospice until very near her death due to the multiple blood transfusions she received. We spent time every week checking labs, ordering blood products, talking of the things she might want to do before she passed away.

The time from diagnosis of acute leukemia to death (especially for someone her age, and especially if it's untreated) is quite short. This can be quite distressing for both patients and families. We "buy them time" with the transfusions. This allows patients time to put things in order. Once they exceed a certain number of transfusions a week, and the leukemia is overwhelming, the patients are usually placed in hospice care.

Her family was very involved. She lived with her granddaughter and great-grandchildren. She had loved to clean house and had been very proud of her home. We would talk of going to a donut shop in a nearby town for lemon-filled donuts. These small pleasures were what made her happy. As her disease progressed, it became more and more difficult for her to do the things she loved. She was forced to walk with a walker. And eventually, she was unable to do much on her own.

As Greta was entering the last days of her life, she became weaker, more fatigued by even the simplest of tasks. During those weekly visits near the end, we had many discussions. I asked her to complete a form, a physician order for life-sustaining treatment, and I asked her to create a durable power of attorney for health care so her family, caregivers, and hospice workers would know her wishes. I spoke at length with her family about some of the behaviors she might exhibit. As her time became shorter, I also talked of the possibility that her husband or another friend or relative might come to her to guide her and go with her.

She was placed in hospice care, as the end of her life was rapidly approaching.

I went to visit her the day prior to her passing. She was in her own room, very weak, her breathing uneven.

Her son pulled me aside to share Greta's bedside story of seeing her husband. As she was nearing death, she reached toward someone she saw whom we could not. She spoke to her husband regarding the next lifetime they might be spending together. She made it clear she didn't want to be a military wife again.

Greta was receiving pain medication for leg and back pain. She was not confused; she was mostly in the next world. She was comfortable. As she moved toward death, her breathing became more labored, and the pain medication was increased. With her symptoms controlled, she was not in distress. She was given medication to help dry the excess secretions, to help decrease or eliminate what many call the "death rattle." The sound from this rattle gives the impression the patient is drowning or is unable to breath.

I received a call the next day—Greta had passed peacefully during the early-morning hours.

While it made them sad to know Greta would no longer be in this life with them, her family was happy she was with her husband, her love, who had preceded her in death.

Preparing the family at the bedside is key. Having open, honest conversations, with guidance and compassion, will prepare them for this most difficult of times.

Pain medication is given not only for pain but to ease the stress of increased respirations and inability to clear secretions from the lungs. Hospice has many options for alleviating symptoms. The focus should be on comfort for the patient during this time. Withholding these much needed medications so the patient will 'wake up' can increase their pain and create increased stress for the patient.

Your experiences and thoughts. How could a situation you have been involved in been improved? What would have made the situation go more smoothly?

_____

_____

_____

_____

_____

_____

_____

_____

_____

_____

_____

_____

_____

_____

_____

_____

_____

_____

Notes

Notes

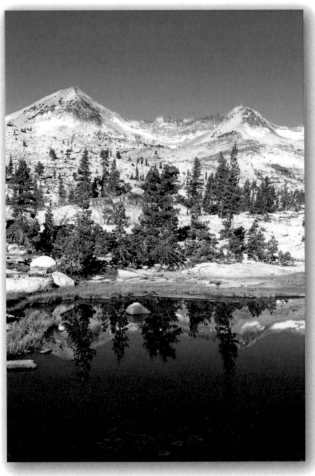

The mountains, magical yet humbling.

Eight

"She was amazing, truly amazing," Danni, my husband at the time, shared with me.

This was how a woman, a magnificent being, was described to me. A week had passed since Danni had been struck by lightning. He finally decided to tell me his story. But let's go back a week in time so I may share more of who this woman was.

"I'm OK," he said, slightly slurring his words.

This is not the first thing you want to hear from your husband at 10:00 p.m. when he is working out of state. Danni was working at a job site near Park City, installing a ski lift.

"I've been hit by lightning, but the doctor says I'll be OK."

Holy cow!

I called the physician at the hospital in Salt Lake City. My concern was his slightly off speech. I was worried he may have sustained injuries due to the intense electrical voltage he had received.

He was, in fact, going to be OK. The lightning entered his right hand and exited his right foot, sparing his heart from the jolt of millions of volts of electricity. He temporarily lost his vision. His right arm and leg were useless as he scrambled off the beam he was standing on. This wooden plank was over the top of a tower footing for a ski lift tower with several of our crew standing in wet concrete below. He said that visually, everything went an eerie, foggy blue. This resolved itself shortly after he crawled to safety. He regained control over his right arm and leg at about the same time. He was taken from the ski slope to Salt Lake City for evaluation. His blood pressure was elevated, but whose wouldn't be!

After the first day or so, a small internal burn presented itself on the ball of his right foot. His jaw was sore for days from the force of it slamming shut due to the intensity of the electricity.

Once his injuries began to improve, Danni called to tell me of a couple of dreams he'd had the night before the lightning strike. He said he was sleeping soundly when he dreamed he was in a "crumpled-up heap" on the ground wearing a yellow rain slicker. He was soaking wet. He was approached by the beautiful woman he'd seen the night before the accident, though not in a sexy way. He described her as truly magnificent even though she was dressed in jeans and a striped shirt. (The angels, or guides, tend to present how the person will most readily receive their visitation.) She walked up, bent down, and kissed his head, and he knew everything would be OK. He awoke from the dream startled. He returned to sleep, only to have the same dream a second time.

When he shared this story with me, I asked about the rain slicker. The lift-building crew wore green or red slickers but not yellow. He said it had started to rain, and as he had just a quarter yard of concrete remaining to pour, he thought he would finish. He ran to the nearest truck and grabbed the slicker off the front seat. It was yellow.

Realizing he'd had an angel visit in his dreams, I asked him if at any time he had thought he would die from the lightning strike.

He hadn't. He knew, even as lightning coursed through his body, he would be OK.

Even with potentially fatal events, there may be a story, a gift of sorts. Danni's angel visits were blessings. To have an angel come to you prior to an accident should be viewed with awe and believed.

With potentially life threatening accidents, most know if they are going to live or die. We have all heard the stories of people having premonitions, the realization their time may be short. Some act strangely, engaging others in deep conversations, visiting people they haven't spent much time with. As we look back to the time prior to someone's death, especially accidents, there are usually clues or events that point towards the person's subconscious knowledge of their impending death.

Your experiences and thoughts. How could a situation you have been involved in been improved? What would have made the situation go more smoothly?

_____

_____

_____

_____

_____

_____

_____

_____

_____

_____

_____

_____

_____

_____

_____

_____

Notes

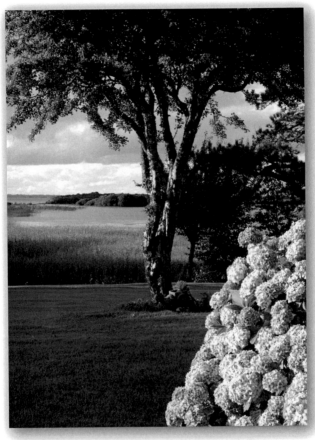

A fairy tree in Ireland. Some believe the
tree is a gateway between worlds.

Nine

"Anna, can you come see me? My family doesn't understand," one of my patients said in a call to me.

Jerry lived just a few miles away and had recently been discharged from the hospital. He was being treated for an illness that eventually would end his life, but it wouldn't be soon.

He did, however, have a serious infection in the hospital and had become septic, which put him into cardiac arrest.

As the medical personnel resuscitated Jerry, he went on a journey. He told me, once he was stable in the ICU, that he knew he had died. He saw the light in the distance. He felt the warmth and love of the world beyond. It was magnificent. All of the cares of his earthbound life melted away. He was filled with so much love, more than he thought was ever possible. As he returned to this life, he was no longer afraid to die.

I went to see him and his family. He appeared to be a bit apprehensive. We stepped into the family room to talk privately.

"My family doesn't understand what I went through. I'm no longer afraid to die. They won't talk with me about how amazing my journey was. They say it scares them. They don't want me to die."

We talked for a couple of hours. We discussed his feelings, what his family must have been going through. They had been there to witness his dying and resuscitation. They were not ready to have him give up. When he expressed he was OK with dying, they felt he did not want to live and had given up hope. They feared he was leaving them.

Months later, he passed away. His family was at his bedside. Not everyone was ready for his death, but there was a sense of peace in the room. Jerry had shown them he was not afraid. He faced his departure from this world with compassion for his family once he was able to verbalize his frustrations.

Patients can feel so alone at this time. Their understanding of life and death has expanded. Change is inevitable for them and their family and friends are not always ready for this change. I suggest heart to heart conversations, even if it scares you. It's a time of growth for everyone.

Not only do the family and friends support and care for the patient, but the dying can also provide insights and support for them. The insights, deep meanings, which come from this time are gifts for us, for those left on earth, while we wait our turn to move on.

Your experiences and thoughts. How could a situation you have been involved in been improved? What would have made the situation go more smoothly?

_____

_____

_____

_____

_____

_____

_____

_____

_____

_____

_____

_____

_____

_____

_____

_____

_____

_____

Notes

Conclusion

The purpose of this book is to give hope: hope that we continue through time in the spiritual lives of our souls. My goals are to provide food for thought and useful information regarding life before and during physical death and regarding the hereafter. I feel so very blessed to work in the field of hematology, oncology, and bone-marrow transplant. My patients are amazing. The insights they have given me compare with no others.

Please contact me via my website, Angelsbythebedside.com, for further information or to book a lecture, ask questions, or share your story. You will find my blog on this site as well. I can also be reached via email at angelsbythebedside@gmail.com. My Facebook page is located under my name, Anna Antonowich.

I wish you blessings for a wonderful day!

Appendix 1:
Definitions of Care

I've included definitions of *home care*, *palliative care*, and *hospice* to help further clarify the services they offer. There is also a small section on pain and pain management.

Home Care

With home care, a registered nurse makes home visits ordered by the health-care provider to evaluate, teach, and monitor patients in the short term, usually until a problem has been resolved or stabilized. Such patients also need to be homebound with the exception of visits to their health-care providers and outings for basic needs.

Palliative Care

Palliative care is another option, similar to home care. To qualify for palliative care, the patient must have a life-limiting illness such as cancer, heart disease, lung disease, or dementia. While receiving palliative care, the patient may continue to receive treatment for their disease that is not curative based, meaning the treatment will not cure the patient. Their treatments are combined with advanced management of pain and other symptoms, with a focus on enhanced quality of life for the patient and family. Palliative care is composed of an inter-disciplinary team of doctors, nurses, social workers, physical therapists, spiritual counselors, dieticians, pharmacists, and other specialists. They provide care uniquely suited for the situation in coordination with the patient's primary care provider and specialists. The palliative-care team assists with navigating the health-care system to optimize care. Emotional and spiritual support is also provided.

Hospice

The shift from active treatment to a focus on quality of life may be difficult for many. When presented with the option of hospice, many feel the patient is "giving up hope" of getting better and may die sooner. The opposite is true. Many patients do better while receiving hospice care than on their own. Hospice care may be provided to patients with a life expectancy of six months or less. Hospice care is designed to make whatever time remains as comfortable and as meaningful as possible. This may include pain control, nursing visits, skilled aides to assist with physical care, and emotional support for the patient, family, and caregivers. Most hospice programs provide grief counseling after the loss of a loved one.

Appendix II: Stages of Dying and Grief

Stages of Dying

Barbara Karnes, RN, put together an amazing set of booklets describing the process leading to the end of life, the dying experience, and grieving after losing a loved one. In her booklet *Gone from My Sight*, I summarized Karnes provides guidelines for the time prior to death, from the weeks to the days to the hours to the minutes before someone passes away.

The months prior to death may be challenging for patients. It's difficult for them to realize life is quickly coming to an end. People will begin to look inward, reflecting on their lives. They will become more fatigued, napping and sleeping more. Conversations are more in depth and may be more spiritual in nature. They watch TV less. Day-to-day routines become less important.

In the weeks before death, patients' appetites wane. As Karnes mentions in *Gone from My Sight*, the body doesn't tolerate food as well as it did before. Meats are the first to be eliminated, then vegetables. These foods take energy to digest, energy that is declining. Meals become smaller, and patients' interest in food declines. Forcing a patient to eat can be distressing for them. I've had patients vomit food because the family became insistent they eat. It can cause patients physical pain to eat and process food. In the days before they die, they eat and drink very little. This is OK. Their bodily systems are slowing down, readying them for physical death. Our society relates food to getting better, to living longer. Not eating feels like a sign patients are giving up.

The dying may also begin seeing loved ones or their "angels," as described earlier in this book. There is a peacefulness that settles around them. At times, they may be distracted by their thoughts and not as engaged with those around them. This can be distressing for family and friends.

Most of those closer to dying will sleep more, have increased fatigued, and will need assistance to move from a chair to the bed or to the shower or to do basic tasks. They will limit visitors, or, if large numbers of people come to visit, they will nap or disengage from them. Speech may become less audible.

Physical changes continue as patients' bodies shut down. They will lose muscle mass and, if the time prior to death is lengthy, will become very thin and cachectic (a condition in which the patient has lost most of their muscle mass, has significant loss of appetite, weakness, loss of weight),. The kidneys begin to shut down. Their urine output decreases, and it becomes darker. There may be increased swelling of the arms and legs due to decreased urinary output. There will also be decreased protein in the blood, causing fluids to push into the tissues. They may not have bowel movements as frequently due to their bowels slowing down from pain medications, inactivity, or dehydration.

There is also a shift in their eyes and the way the eyes look. Their eyes will be distant and vacant. I believe there is a blending of worlds during this time. One foot is with us, and the other in the hereafter.

In the hours prior to death, the dying may not be aroused easily. Breathing will become erratic, or patients may experience Cheyne-Stokes breathing, with periods of apnea followed by increased respirations that ramp up, then quickly decline. They may "guppy breathe," similar to how fish gulp when they are out of water. Because they cannot breathe or cough deeply to clear secretions from their lungs and throat, what has been called a "death rattle" may occur. This may sound as though they are drowning, but they aren't. Medications can dry up these secretions. This is not as distressing for the patient as it is for the loved ones at the bedside.

At the time of physical death, patients will stop breathing. The pulse will slow and then stop. Their hands and feet may already be cool or cold to the touch, their legs slightly mottled in color. Their trunk or upper arms may still be warm, but the flow of blood will have stopped. Their mouth may remain open. At times, one or two delayed last breaths will be expelled, catching those at the bedside by surprise.

During these last few days, while patients may not be able to respond or continue to talk with their loved ones, the last sense to leave is their hearing. Withholding pain medication or sedation so a family member can "wake them up" may be cruel and cause the patient more pain and distress. I always recommend those at the bedside continue to talk even as patients take their last breaths—and even as the bodies are cleaned and readied to be taken away.

Grief

Elizabeth Kubler-Ross discusses the "stages" or experiences of grieving in her book *On Death and Dying*. The reason "stages" is placed in quotations is because her book was based not on scientific research but on observations from the bedsides of thousands of patients near the end of their lives. She found there were similarities in how the dying deal with the emotional states surrounding impending death. Her book focuses on the importance of listening to the dying. So the "stages" are meant to facilitate discussions and provide guidance rather than to manage dying patients.

When someone is told of a terminal illness, a condition or disease expected to take his or her life, the person will likely experience various emotional states. The length of time of each stage varies from person to person. At times, someone will have a blurring of these stages. Kubler-Ross discusses the stages of denial, anger, bargaining, depression, and acceptance.

When first receiving a diagnosis, a person may experience shock.

Overlapping these stages is hope, which begins soon after prognosis and continues until death. Hope should never be discouraged or taken away from patients. What will change, though, is what they are hoping for. Some may hope initially for a misdiagnosis thus changing their prognosis. Or they may hope a cure will be found to prolong their lives. As they realize life will come to an end at some point, they will hope their pain will be in control or that they won't die alone.

Kubler-Ross also wrote *On Life after Death*, in which she discusses the continuum from this life into the next. She defines spirituality not as based on religion but as a knowing, that there is something far greater than we are.

In her book she talks of three stages of death, which she likens to a cocoon and a butterfly. The shedding of the cocoon is part of the life of the butterfly. Death does not exist as the end of everything as many believe. Kubler-Ross was told by the people she met with of the bodily wholeness they felt, just as someone might continue to feel a lost limb.

Kubler-Ross also encourages using her book to spark conversations. It was meant to expose readers, the loved ones at the bedside, and the dying to another way of viewing this experience as I am attempting with this book. By reading the stories of others, a common bond is recognized, and may be acted upon, with knowing others have been in a similar situation.

Appendix III: Pain

Pain can vary in intensity from mild to extreme. Patients can rate their pain to let their doctors and family know what they are feeling. It is a subjective rating. A pain scale of zero to ten, with ten being the most extreme, is the most common method of rating pain. Adequate pain management is essential.

The causes of pain are not always physical. People may experience spiritual, emotional, psychological, or social pain related to their disease. Physical pain may be increased by stressors brought about by emotional, social, or psychological pain. Other symptoms such as nausea and vomiting, constipation, diarrhea, or shortness of breath may also be related to pain, thus increasing distress.

Control of pain is essential for enhancing the quality of life as someone nears the end of life. Living in pain may prevent the dying from experiencing a peaceful and comfortable death

After a loved one has passed, if stressful situations have occurred, those left behind may have guilt and painful memories,

References

Karnes, Barbara. 1984. *Gone from My Sight: The Dying Experience*. Vancouver: Barbara Karnes Books, Inc.

Kubler-Ross, E. 1969. *On Death and Dying*. New York: The Macmillan Company.

Kubler-Ross, E. 1991. *On Life after Death*. Berkeley: Celestial Arts.

Resources

American Cancer Society

www.cancer.org

ACS, American Cancer Society, is an organization which provides medical information related to cancer diagnoses, their treatment and care. They also provide resources for patients, families and health care providers.

CaringBridge

Caringbridge.org

Caringbridge provides an online format and web site for patients, families and friends to connect with each other to provide support and information.

Aging with Dignity: The Five Wishes (guidance and documents for the end of life) https://www.agingwithdignity.org/five-wishes/about-five-wishes

A document which provides not only Durable Power of Attorney for Healthcare, but provides the patient a chance to be more specific with things such as what music would they like played at the bedside prior to their passing away, what would they like their friends and family to know for example.

Livestrong
Livestrong.org
Provides support information and resources for patients with cancer.

National Caregivers Library
www.caregiverslibrary.org
An organization which provides caregivers with a multitude of resource information related to caregiving and for seniors.

Made in the USA
San Bernardino, CA
13 January 2018